I0790276

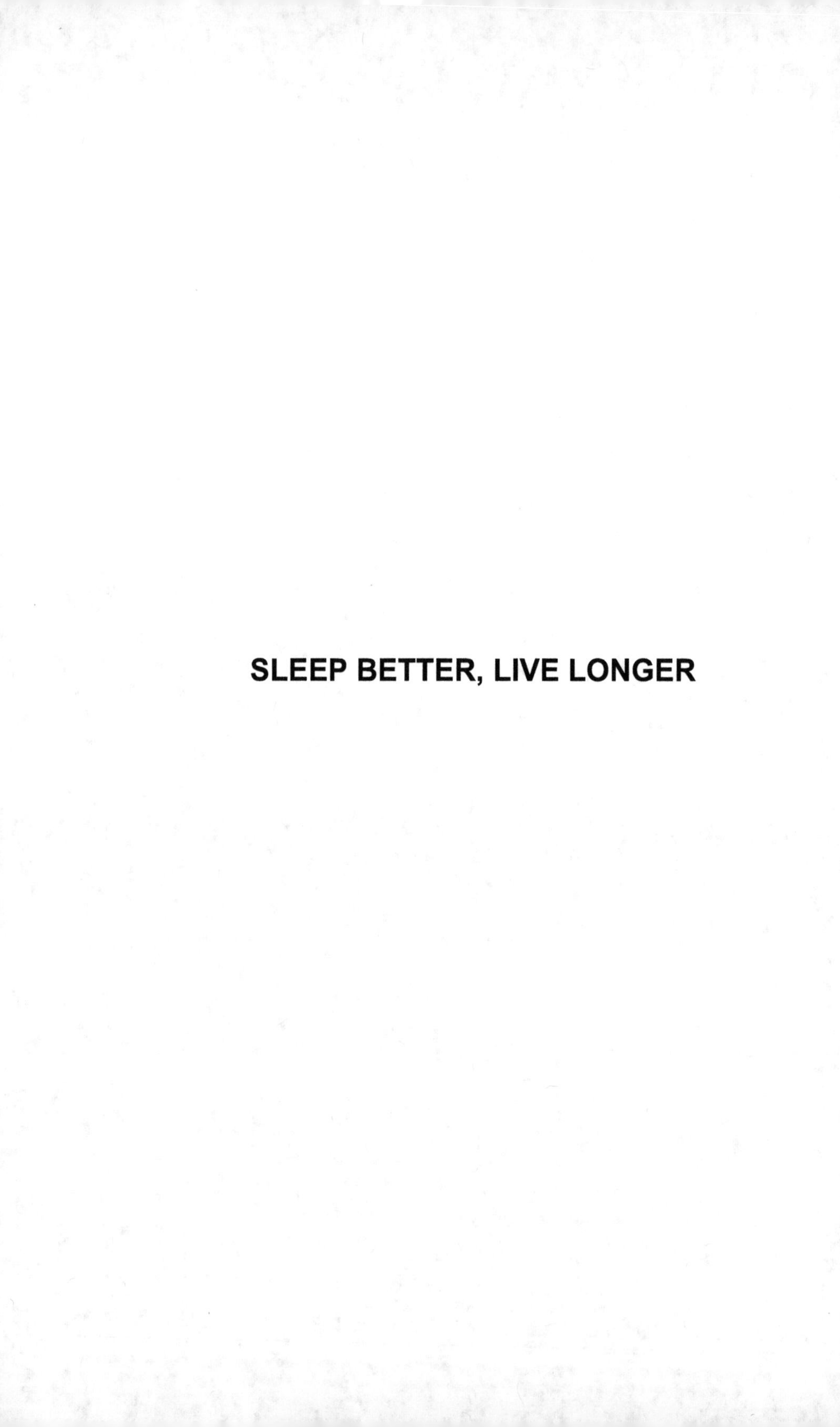

SLEEP BETTER, LIVE LONGER

SLEEP BETTER, LIVE LONGER

THE VITAL ROLE OF REST IN HEART HEALTH

DR. ALBERT THOMPSON

DEDICATION

To everyone who wants to be healthier and happier, may you find the strength to put your rest first. Because every deep sleep holds the promise of a healthy heart and a longer life.

To my patients, whose stories inspire me every day. You have taught me that getting enough sleep can often light the way to health.

Thank you for telling me of how important balance and self-care are to my family, whose love and support keep me motivated to heal.

Thank you for reading this book. May we all understand how important rest is and may our hearts get stronger with each quiet night.

Dr. Albert Thompson

TABLE OF CONTENTS

INTRODUCTION

Why Good Sleep Is Important for Heart Health

As a doctor who has studied the human body for decades, I have seen people get better after being close to dying. Sleep is one thing I've always been surprised by how little attention it gets. It's what everything is built on. People often think that we give up sleep to be more productive or because of how busy life is these days. Still, the truth is that sleep is the body's main way of healing, especially the heart.

Let me tell you about Michael. He was one of the first patients I ever had. At 45 years old, he was a business leader who looked like he was living the dream. But his heart was hurting inside. Michael had been having problems with high blood pressure and cholesterol, but even though he was taking medicine and making changes to his lifestyle, his health wasn't getting better.

What did he not have? Rest. He told them that he only slept four to five hours a night because he had so much to do and work to do.

Michael's health got a lot better after he made sleep a priority by working with a sleep specialist and following a good sleep hygiene practice. His heart function got better, his blood pressure went back to normal, and his energy level went back to where it had been ten years ago. His case is a strong warning of how important sleep is for the most important organ in the body.

The Important Link Between Rest and Living Longer

Your heart can slow down and start over when you sleep. Although the heart beats nonstop all day, it needs breaks to work at its best. Think of sleep as your body's natural way of fixing itself. Your heart rate slows down, your blood pressure levels off, and your body does important repairs. This rest is very important for keeping the heart and lungs healthy.

New studies regularly show that not getting enough sleep (defined as less than seven hours per night) greatly raises the risk of heart disease, stroke, and even dying too soon. Studies have shown that getting enough good sleep can make you live longer by lowering these risks. What matters is not how much sleep you get, but how well you sleep. Sleep problems, like sleep apnea, can keep the heart from getting the rest it needs, which can hurt it over time.

Why Getting Enough Good Sleep is Important for Heart Health

There is no question that sleep and heart health are linked. As you get deeper into sleep, your blood valves loosen up, which makes it easier for your heart to pump. Getting the right mix of hormones while you sleep helps keep inflammation, stress, and heart health in check. If you can't do this because of insomnia, chronic lack of sleep, or a sleep problem, your heart will suffer.

As a doctor, I tell my patients that they should take sleep just as seriously as they do food and exercise. The third important part of health that people often forget about is sleep. Think of your heart as an engine. Even the best engines break down if they aren't taken care of properly. That upkeep comes from sleep, which gives your heart the rest it needs to work well.

This is true, as shown by Michael's story. He not only made his heart healthier, but he also made his life better. His story is similar to that of thousands of other people who have found that sleep can change their lives. It's not time lost when you sleep; it's time spent on your health, your heart, and your future.

I'll explain the science behind the link between sleep and heart health in this book, along with some useful tips for making both better. Get some rest and take care of your heart, which is the most important organ in your body.

CHAPTER 1

Understanding Sleep's Role in Cardiovascular Health

As a cardiologist, I've had the chance to work with people who have heart disease at different stages. One question I ask almost all of my new patients is, "How well are you sleeping?" People are often caught off guard by this question. But the truth is that sleep is much more important for heart health than most people think.

I want to tell you a story about Laura, a 50 years old woman who came to see me because she had been having chest pains. She worked out often, ate well, and was in good shape. At first glance, her way of life looked great. Even though she had all the right habits, she had high blood pressure and early signs of heart disease.

After a run of tests ruled out other possibilities, we looked into her routine more. Laura thought her busy schedule didn't allow for more sleep, so she only got about five hours of sleep each night. We found that the one thing she wasn't doing getting enough sleep was really hurting her heart.

How Sleep Affects the Heart's Ability to Work

Your body doesn't just shut down while you sleep, it works to heal and renew itself. Sleep is a time for your heart to rest and heal. There are times during sleep when your heart rate slows down and blood pressure drops.

This gives your heart a much needed break. This is like your heart's "rest and digest" mode.

But not getting enough sleep or getting bad sleep puts your heart under ongoing stress. If you don't get enough sleep, your heart doesn't have time to fully heal from the stresses of the day. This can cause long-term high blood pressure, more inflammation, and a higher chance of heart disease and stroke. Studies have shown that people who sleep less than six hours a night are more likely to get heart problems than people who sleep seven to eight hours a night.

Laura's chest pains went away and her blood pressure slowly went down once she started to make sleep a priority. For some reason, she didn't think that sleep was important for her heart health.

The Science Behind Sleep That Heals

Sleep is not just something you do while you're not doing anything, it's a biologically complicated process that fixes the body's systems. Sleep is very important for keeping the respiratory system working well. Your body releases growth hormone when you get into deeper stages of sleep. This hormone helps repair organs, like the heart and blood vessels.

Restorative sleep also helps keep chemicals like adrenaline and cortisol in check, which affects heart rate and blood pressure. When these hormones are out of whack because you didn't get enough sleep, it can cause your stress response to be too strong, which puts extra stress on your heart.

It's during these deep moments of sleep that the heart gets the rest it needs. During this time off, the body fixes inflammation and keeps blood sugar levels stable, which are both important for lowering the risk of heart disease.

What Stages of Sleep Do to Your Heart Health?

We need to look at the different stages of sleep to fully understand how sleep affects the heart. As you sleep, your eyes move quickly back and forth between three non-REM stages and one REM state.

- **Stage 1 of NREM:** This is the lightest stage of sleep, when you come and go from being awake. It's the change from being awake to asleep. It's important, but it doesn't have a big effect on the heart.

- **NREM Stage 2:** Your body temperature drops and your heart rate starts to slow down in this stage. This is the first break for the heart, and you spend about half of your sleep in this stage.

- **NREM Stage 3 (Deep Sleep):** The heart rate and blood pressure are the lowest during this part of sleep, which is meant to help you heal. During this stage, the heart fully recovers, and the body works hard to fix cells, lower inflammation, and keep important things in check, like blood sugar and cholesterol levels. Heart health depends on getting enough deep sleep.

- **REM sleep:** This is the dream phase of sleep. During REM, your heart rate goes up a little, but this stage is very important for keeping your emotions in check and forming memories. Both of these things help you deal with stress and keep your heart healthy.

All of these steps are important for keeping your heart healthy. Skipping any of them or not getting enough of them, especially deep sleep, can put stress on the heart over time.

I've seen this many times before, but Laura's case made it clearer, it's not how many hours you sleep that counts, but

Dr. Albert Thompson

how well you sleep. Putting sleep first isn't just about feeling refreshed, it also helps protect your heart and makes you live longer.

The Hidden Dangers of Not Getting Enough Sleep

A few years ago, I saw a man named David in my office. He was 52 years old and had never had heart disease before, but he was having sudden chest pain, shortness of breath, and tiredness. David couldn't figure out why his health was quickly getting worse even though he ate well and worked out daily. I asked him about his sleep after a number of tests cleared out common heart problems. David had been getting by on just five hours of sleep every night for years because he was sure he could handle his busy life without giving up time for work or family. He didn't know it, but not getting enough sleep was putting a lot of stress on his heart.

David's situation is not at all unusual. Lack of sleep is an unseen threat to heart health that a lot of people, including him, don't see. This chapter will talk about how not getting enough sleep can hurt your heart. It will also talk about common sleep problems that come with big risks, as well as the early warning signs you should look out for before things get worse.

Dr. Albert Thompson

What Happens to Your Heart When You Don't Get Enough Sleep?

When it comes to the heart, not getting enough sleep can be a quiet killer. Our bodies go into a recovery mode while we sleep. Our blood pressure drops, our heart rate slows, and the heart and blood vessels fix themselves very quickly. This time for healing is cut short when you don't get enough sleep, which can cause your blood pressure, heart rate, and inflammation to rise. These effects add up over time, making heart disease, stroke, and even heart failure more likely.

People like David who don't get enough sleep on a regular basis may have higher amounts of stress hormones like adrenaline and cortisol, which make the heart work harder than it should. The body's "fight or flight" reaction is set off by these hormones. This makes the person constantly alert, which wears down the cardiovascular system.

Not getting enough sleep not only has a direct effect on the heart, but it also makes it harder for your body to control blood sugar, which can lead to insulin resistance. This makes you more likely to get type 2 diabetes, which is another major cause of heart disease.

In the case of David, his chest pains and tiredness slowly went away after we helped him change the way he slept.

His story is a strong reminder that sleep is more than just a break from your day, it's important for your heart health and general health.

Common Sleep Disorders and the Heart Risks They Possess

Many times, not getting enough sleep is due to a sleep problem, but many people don't know they have one. Let us look at some of the most common sleep problems and how they make heart health worse.

- **Apnea while you sleep:** This is one of the worst sleep problems for the heart. People with sleep apnea have trouble breathing while they sleep because their mouth gets blocked. The oxygen level drops during these breaks in breathing, which can last from a few seconds to a minute. Blood pressure goes up because the heart has to work harder to get fresh blood to all parts of the body. If sleep apnea isn't treated, the chance of heart attacks, strokes, high blood pressure, and irregular heartbeats goes up over time.

- **Trouble sleeping:** Sleep apnea may seem worse than insomnia, but long-term sleeplessness can be just as bad for your heart health. People who have trouble sleeping are often very stressed and anxious, which can make their blood pressure and heart rate stay high for a long time. Studies have shown that people who have trouble sleeping are more likely to get heart disease and high blood pressure.

- **Restless Leg Syndrome (RLS):** Even though RLS mostly affects the legs, it can also have an effect on the heart. The constant need to move the legs, which is often painful, can make it very hard to sleep. People who have RLS may find it hard to get into deeper stages of sleep, which keeps their heart from getting the full rest it needs. In the long run, this broken sleep can lead to problems with the heart.

- **Narcolepsy:** This is a neurological disease that causes people to be sleepy all the time and have sudden sleep attacks. It can also be bad for your heart health. Narcolepsy is not very common, but it can mess up your usual sleep patterns and cause heart problems because your sleep-wake cycles are off and your sleep quality is bad overall.

Finding Early Warning Signs of Heart Problems Caused by Sleep Loss

Heart problems caused by lack of sleep don't always show clear symptoms, but there are signs you can look out for to make sure your heart doesn't get seriously hurt. If you know these early warning signs, you can get medical help before things get worse.

✓ **Headaches in the morning**

People who have sleep apnea often wake up with headaches because their bodies didn't get enough air while they were sleeping. This could be an early sign that your heart is beating too fast at night

✓ **Daytime fatigue that can't be explained**

If you feel very tired during the day, even after what seems like a full night's sleep, it could mean that the quality of your sleep is bad. If you feel tired all the time, it's likely that you're not getting enough restful sleep, which can put stress on your heart over time.

✓ **Staying awake at night a lot**

If you often wake up in the middle of the night for no reason, it could mean you have a sleep problem like sleep apnea. Each awakening throws off the usual flow of sleep stages, which keeps your heart from going into its healing mode.

✓ **Pain in the chest or heart palpitations at night**

If you feel pain or your heart beats irregularly while you sleep, you should get medical help right away. These could be signs of high blood pressure or other heart problems that are linked to not getting enough sleep.

Dr. Albert Thompson

✓ Snoring and gasping for air

A clear sign of sleep apnea is loud snoring followed by quiet, gasping for air, or choking for air. It's very important to see a doctor if you or someone you know has these signs.

This story about David teaches us a valuable lesson, skipping sleep can have bad effects on your heart. Many people with similar symptoms don't know that the way they sleep could be hurting their heart in a silent way. We need to start thinking of sleep as the important part of heart health that it is.

By learning about the secret risks of not getting enough sleep, we can protect our hearts and live healthier lives.

CHAPTER 3

Stress, Sleep, and Heart Health

Marcus was one of my patients. He was a high level businessman in his early 40s. Marcus was driven, successful, and used to dealing with the stress of his job. But in the past few months, he had started having bothersome symptoms, such as high blood pressure, headaches, and chest pain that would wake him up in the middle of the night. Marcus didn't seem like the typical person who would get heart disease, but his stress was making it hard for him to sleep and hurting his heart.

After doing tests, it was clear that his worry was having a big effect on his heart. Even worse was the fact that he was sleeping in strange places. When Marcus was awake, his mind would race with work thoughts for hours on end. He would then fall asleep for short periods of time. It was very clear that worry, lacking sleep, and heart health are all linked. Marcus's heart health got a lot better after we started helping him deal with his stress and get better sleep.

Dr. Albert Thompson

How Stress Affects the Quality of Sleep and How Well the Heart Works

Worry is a normal reaction to problems, but long-term worry, especially the kind that keeps you up at night, can hurt your heart. Hormones like adrenaline and cortisol are released by your body when you're stressed. These hormones speed up your heart rate and raise your blood pressure. This is part of your body's "fight or flight" reaction, which is meant to keep you safe when you're in danger. But when this response happens over and over again because of worry, it puts pressure on the heart all the time.

Stress makes it harder to fall asleep and stay asleep. The more stressed you are, the harder it is to fall asleep and stay asleep. That's because the stress hormone cortisol makes it hard to calm down and get into deep, healing sleep. Your body doesn't calm down when you try to sleep. Instead, it stays alert all the time. Not getting enough sleep makes you more stressed, which makes you sleep worse, which makes your heart work harder.

Stress also has a direct effect on your heart health by making your blood vessels more inflamed, which raises your chance of heart disease and plaque buildup. Stress hormones that are always present can cause high blood pressure, irregular heart beats, and other heart problems over time.

Getting out of the Stress Sleep Cycle

Stopping the stress sleep cycle is important for saving your heart and getting better sleep. In Marcus's case, we worked together to figure out what was making him stressed and how to deal with it. This helped him recover control of his heart health and sleep.

To break this cycle, you must first understand how your body reacts to worry. Do you often stay up at night worried about things you need to do or the future? Do you notice that stress makes it harder for you to sleep at certain times of the year? Once you know what causes your stress, you can start to deal with it before it gets worse.

After that, it's important to stick to a regular sleep schedule. When you go to bed and wake up at the same time every day, you're more likely to get a good night's sleep without any interruptions. This is very important for lowering your stress and letting your heart rest.

Making a "wind-down" process that tells your body it's time to go into sleep mode is another important step. For example, slow breathing, meditation, or light stretching can be used to help calm the nervous system before bed. Marcus started doing breathing exercises and reading a book that had nothing to do with work every night. This helped calm his mind and get his body ready for sleep.

How to Deal with Stress to Sleep Better

Taking care of your stress well can protect your heart and help you sleep better. Here are some tried and true ways to lower stress and get a good night's sleep:

- **Being mindful and meditating:** Meditation and other mindfulness techniques are great ways to lower stress. By focusing on the present, mindfulness helps to calm the mind and stop thoughts from rushing. This makes it easier to go to sleep. Regular mindfulness practice has been shown to drop cortisol levels and make sleep better.

  Focusing on your breathing is a simple way to practice awareness. Close your eyes, find a nice place to sit, and take slow, deep breaths. Count to four as you breathe in, hold for one second, and then slowly breathe out for another four counts. Before going to bed, do this five to ten times to calm your thought.

- **Progressive Muscle Relaxation (RMR):** By systematically tensing and relaxing different groups of muscles in your body, this method can help you get rid of the stress-related tension that builds up in your body. To begin, tense your toes and hold for five seconds. Then, slowly let go. Move up through your body calves, legs, stomach, chest, arms, and shoulders until you feel fully relaxed.

- **Do regular exercise:** One of the best ways to deal with worry is to do something active. Your body releases endorphins when you work out. These are natural stress breakers that make you feel better and lower your cortisol levels. But do not work out hard right before bed, as it might keep you awake. Instead, try to do some moderate exercise early in the day to help you sleep well.

- **Make your environment sleep-friendly:** The place where you sleep has a lot to do with how well you rest. Because these things help you sleep, make sure your bedroom is dark, quiet, and cool. Also, get rid of any electronics or other things that might be stimulating to your brain before bed.

- **Don't drink too much alcohol or caffeine:** Even though a glass of wine might sound like a good way to relax, it can get in the way of deep sleep. If you eat or drink something with caffeine in it too close to bedtime, it can keep you awake. Caffeine is found in coffee, tea, and chocolate. Cutting back on these things in the evening can help your body calm down naturally before bed.

- **Writing:** It can help to clear your mind to write down your thoughts before bed. A lot of people find that writing down their worries or to-do lists in a book helps them "offload" their stress, which makes them feel better and ready to sleep. Marcus found this method to be especially helpful for dealing with stress at work.

Marcus's trip showed me how much stress can hurt your heart and your ability to sleep. Once he started using the above techniques to deal with his worry, both his sleep and his heart health got a lot better. He no longer had chest pains, his blood pressure stayed the same, and he felt more energy during the day.

To take charge of your health and break the harmful loop that many of us are stuck in, you need to understand the link between stress, sleep, and heart function. Stress is a normal part of life, but if you know how to handle it well, you can keep your heart healthy and sleep better.

CHAPTER 4

Getting Better Sleep to Make Your Heart Stronger

Linda, a 55-year-old woman who had always been a night owl and one of my patients, came to see me because she was constantly tired and worried about her heart health. No matter how hard she tried to stay busy, she often felt tired and cranky during the day. She was having trouble sleeping, which was affecting both her energy levels and her heart health. This became clear after a long conversation.

One important thing that Linda's case makes clear is something that many of us forget, good sleep habits is one of the most important things for heart health. Everyday habits can either help us sleep well or keep us from sleeping well, and these habits can have long-lasting effects on the health and resilience of our hearts.

Sleep Hygiene, Daily Habits that will Help You Sleep Better

Linda had always thought that on the weekends she could "make up" for lost sleep. But I told her that our bodies work best when they are consistent, and that sleeping at odd times can mess up our circadian rhythm, which is our natural sleep wake cycle and is important for keeping our hearts healthy.

21

Dr. Albert Thompson

Setting up good sleep habits is the key to better sleep quality and, by default, better heart health. Sleep hygiene is the set of daily habits and actions that help you get good, restful sleep. Linda was able to fall asleep faster and stay asleep longer after making a few small changes to her habit. This had a huge effect on her health and happiness.

For better sleep health, here are some steps you can take right now:

- **Maintain a Regular Sleep Schedule:** Your body's internal clock works better when you go to bed and wake up at the same time every day. Aim for 7–9 hours of sleep every night, and don't give in to the urge to make big changes to your routine on the weekends. Linda felt better and more awake during the day after setting a regular time to go to bed and wake up.

- **Develop a Calming Pre-Sleep Routine:** Engaging in relaxing activities before bed sends to your brain that it's time to wind down. You could read a book, listen to soothing music, or do some gentle yoga moves. Linda found that meditating for 20 minutes before bed helped her calm down and stop her mind from running.

- **Limit Screen Time Before Bed:** The blue light that phones, tablets, and computers give off can stop your body from making melatonin, a hormone that controls sleep. Stay away from screens for at least an hour before bed, and do something relaxing that isn't digital instead.

Making a Sleep Environment That Is Good for Your Heart

Another place where small changes made a big difference was Linda's bedroom. With the TV on in the background, she thought it would help her fall asleep. But when she learned that light and noise from outside can make it hard to sleep, she chose to make her bedroom a place where she could relax.

For good sleep, you need a sleep setting that is good for your heart. To make one, follow these steps:

- **Make sure your bedroom is cool and dark:** The darkness tells your body it's time to sleep. Buy blackout shades to keep the room cool (between 60 and 67°F/15 and 19°C) and block out any outside light. This will help you sleep deeply and without interruptions.
- **Limit Noise and Distractions:** If you live in a noisy area, you might want to use earplugs or a white noise machine to block out sounds that are

bothersome. As you fall deeper into sleep, you need to be quiet for your heart rate to slow down.

- **Pick out a smooth mattress and pillows:** The amount of comfort you have has a direct effect on how well you sleep. Make sure that your mattress gives your body enough support and that your pillows keep your neck and back in the right place. Linda bought a new mattress, and right away she could tell that it helped her sleep better.

- **Take away all electronics:** Keeping your phone or TV out of the bedroom can help your brain remember that it's only for sleeping and not for work or fun. She found that making her bedroom a tech-free zone helped her sleep better and fall asleep faster.

The Role of Nutrition and Exercise in Sleep Quality

Linda's road to better sleep didn't end with her bedtime routine or her bedroom environment. We also looked closely at what she ate and how much she worked out. Both of these things have a big effect on how well you sleep, which in turn has an effect on how good your heart is.

A healthy food can make all the difference when it comes to getting a good night's sleep. Different foods and drinks can make it harder to fall asleep, while others can help you relax and sleep better.

✓ **Don't drink or eat anything stimulating before bed**

Caffeine, which is found in coffee, tea, chocolate, and some sweets, can stay in your body for hours and make it hard to fall asleep. The same is true for alcohol, it may make you feel sleepy, but it can wake you up in the middle of the night during deep sleep stages. Limiting your caffeine and drink intake in the hours before bed will help you sleep better.

✓ **Eat foods that help you sleep**

Foods that are high in serotonin, magnesium, and melatonin can help you calm down and fall asleep faster. Some of these are leafy green veggies, bananas, turkey, and almonds. Having a small snack of these things before bed can help you sleep better.

✓ **Exercise regularly, but do it at the right time**

Exercise is good for your heart and can help you sleep better by lowering your stress and making you feel more relaxed. However, doing a lot of intense exercise right before bed can keep you awake and unable to fall asleep. As much as possible, work out early in the day. This will help you sleep better at night.

Dr. Albert Thompson

Linda's life changed when she started going for walks in the morning and changed her diet by cutting back on caffeine and booze. Not only did she say she felt more rested, but she also said she noticed changes in her heart health.

Linda's story shows how simple changes to your living can make a big difference in your heart health and sleep. You can set yourself up for long-term cardiovascular health by learning about the value of daily habits like good sleep hygiene, making your environment restful, and making healthier choices about food and exercise.

CHAPTER 5

Sleep Solutions for Heart Patients

Michael, a 62-year-old man with a history of heart disease, was one of my long-term patients. I remember him very well. Michael was trying to eat well and work out regularly to keep his heart healthy, but he was having trouble sleeping. He would gasp for air several times a night when he woke up, and he was always tired during the day. There was clearly more going on than just normal sleeplessness. Michael was diagnosed with sleep apnea after some tests. If this disease is not treated, it greatly raises the risk of heart problems

Michael's story is not the only one like it. A lot of people with heart problems have trouble sleeping. The good news is that there are ways to help. It can make all the difference to know what to do differently for heart patients and work closely with their doctors.

Some things people with heart conditions should think about when they sleep

For people who already have heart problems, sleep isn't just about feeling relaxed the next day, it also keeps the heart from getting worse. Heart disease and sleep problems often go together, and one can make the other worse. Some health problems, like congestive heart failure, atrial fibrillation, or high blood pressure, can make it hard to sleep. Not getting enough sleep can also put more stress on the heart.

Michael had sleep apnea, which is a common sleep problem that can make heart health worse. People with sleep apnea stop breathing many times while they sleep, which lowers the amount of oxygen in their blood. This puts a lot of stress on the heart and blood vessels, which raises the chance of heart attacks and strokes and makes heart failure worse.

It's important to sleep differently if you have a heart problem. Here are some extra things to think about:

- **Keep an eye out for signs at night:** People with heart problems should pay extra attention to chest pain, shortness of breath, or irregular heartbeats at night. These could be signs of more major problems with sleep.

- **Think about your sleeping position:** People who have heart failure or other heart problems may feel better and breathe better if they sleep on their side or in a raised position. Using pillows to prop yourself up or a movable bed can be helpful.

- **Know the Position of Medicines:** Some heart medicines can impact sleep by either making it impossible to sleep or making you sleep too much. If you think your drugs are making it hard for you to sleep, talk to your doctor about changing them.

Taking Care of Sleep Apnea, Insomnia, and Other Conditions

Sleep apnea is a common problem for people with heart disease, as Michael's story shows. But this isn't the only sleep condition that can be dangerous. Other conditions, like insomnia and restless legs syndrome, can also make it hard to sleep and hurt your heart health.

- **Sleep Apnea**

The most popular way to treat sleep apnea is with Continuous Positive Airway Pressure (CPAP). This machine keeps your lungs open and makes sure you breathe properly all night by sending a steady stream of air through a mask. Michael started using a CPAP machine, and within a few weeks, he woke up less often at night and felt less tired during the day. More importantly, his heart health got better, which made it less likely that he would have problems again.

- **Insomnia**

Not getting enough sleep on a regular basis can make you more stressed, raise your blood pressure, and even lead

Dr. Albert Thompson

to heart disease. Cognitive Behavioral Therapy for Insomnia (CBT-I) and other behavioral treatments can help heart patients a lot. This therapy helps people change their bad thoughts about sleep and start sleeping better.

- **Restless Legs Syndrome (RLS)**

This is a condition that makes it hard to fall asleep because it makes your legs feel bad, especially at night. If you have heart disease and don't treat RLS, you might not get enough sleep, which can make your heart disease worse. In Michael's case, we made sure that his RLS was handled by making changes to his lifestyle, like getting more iron, and giving him medicines that helped ease his symptoms.

- **Circadian Rhythm Disorders**

Heart patients who have trouble sleeping regularly, like shift workers or people who get jet lag, may have problems with their circadian rhythm, which is the body's normal sleep-wake cycle. This can make you more likely to get heart disease over time. Trying to stick to the same sleep plan every night, even on the weekends, can help keep your circadian rhythms in check and improve your heart health.

Working with health care professionals to get better sleep

One of the most important things Michael did to fix his sleep problems was to work closely with his med team. Heart patients often need help from more than one professional to deal with sleep problems. Heart doctors, sleep doctors, and general care doctors can work together to make a treatment plan that takes care of both heart health and sleep quality.

- **Comprehensive Sleep Evaluations**

You should ask your doctor about a sleep study if you think you might have a sleep problem. You can learn a lot about how well you're sleeping and whether you have conditions like sleep apnea by doing this. Michael had a sleep study that proved he had sleep apnea and led to his life-changing CPAP treatment.

- **Changes to your medications**

Some heart medicines can make it hard to sleep, while others can help you sleep better. You can get better sleep without hurting your heart by working with your doctor to change your medications. This could mean taking them at different times of the day or moving to different ones.

- **Lifestyle Changes**

Michael found that making easy changes to his routine, like not eating or drinking heavy meals before bed and doing relaxing things like reading, helped him relax before bed and feel more rested in the morning.

- **Follow-Up Care**

People with sleep problems often need to be managed over time. By seeing your doctor on a regular basis, you can make sure that any treatments, like CPAP therapy, are working well and that your heart condition stays stable.

Michael went from being tired all the time and having problems with his heart health to sleeping better and getting his energy back. This was a strong reminder of how important sleep is for heart patients. Heart patients can improve not only their sleep but also their general heart health by getting help for sleep disorders early on and working closely with their doctors.

CHAPTER 6

How Better Sleep Leads to a Healthier and Longer Life

Working as a doctor for many years, I've seen many people go through big changes just by putting sleep first. Sarah, a 48 years old woman with high blood pressure who was starting to show signs of early heart disease, is one case that stands out. Her health wasn't getting better as fast as we had thought, even though she was taking medicine and making some changes to her lifestyle. She was stressed out, busy, and most importantly, she wasn't sleeping well. She told me that she had been only getting five hours of sleep every night for years.

Sarah agreed to work on getting better sleep after we talked for a long time about how sleep affects heart health. We worked together to make a sleep plan that included better sleep habits, ways to relax, and ways to deal with her stress. The changes were big in just a few months. Sarah's heart health got better, her energy came back, and her blood pressure went down. It was clear, getting enough good sleep was what was missing.

Dr. Albert Thompson

How Getting More Sleep can Help you Live Longer and Healthier

During sleep, the body goes through important changes that directly affect heart health and life. Your heart rate slows down and blood pressure drops while you sleep. This gives your circulatory system time to heal and rebuild. These times of rest every night help lower the risk of getting heart disease and make things better for people who already have heart problems.

- **Better Blood Pressure:** One of the best things about getting enough sleep is that it lowers blood pressure. One of the main reasons people get heart disease is having hypertension, or consistently high blood pressure. Your blood pressure goes down when you sleep well. This gives your heart and blood vessels a break from the steady pressure they feel during the day. Over time, getting enough sleep can lower your blood pressure and lower your risk of having a heart attack or stroke.

- **Lower Inflammation:** Not getting enough sleep on a regular basis makes inflammation worse in the body, which is a major cause of atherosclerosis, the narrowing of the arteries that can cause heart attacks. Your body makes fewer stress chemicals and inflammatory markers when you get enough restful sleep. This helps keep your arteries healthy and flexible.

- **Good for your metabolism and weight control:** Not getting enough sleep makes it more likely that you will have trouble controlling your weight, and being overweight is a major risk factor for heart disease. Hormones that control hunger and metabolism are helped to work better by sleep. Not getting enough sleep makes you hungry and makes you want high-calorie, high fat foods, which can make you gain weight. You can better control your metabolism, stay at a healthy weight, and ease stress on your heart by getting better sleep.

Success Stories: Real-Life Examples of How Heart Health Can Change

Sarah's story is not the only one like it. I've seen a huge number of people whose heart health improved dramatically after getting enough good sleep. Sleep is an important part of long-term health, from correcting early signs of heart disease to getting better after heart surgery. Take a look at these more success stories from people who got better sleep

Carlos, 55 years old: Carlos had trouble sleeping and thinking straight after a heart attack, which slowed his healing. He was able to sleep well again after learning relaxation methods and making changes to his bedroom. His heart function got a lot better on follow-up tests, and he got back the energy and strength he had lost after his heart attack.

Linda, age 63: Linda was always tired and stressed after being diagnosed with Atrial Fibrillation (AFib). Her heart beats weren't normal, which made it hard for her to sleep well. Linda's AFib episodes went down when she started CPAP therapy and made changes to her lifestyle that helped her sleep. Her general heart health also got a lot better.

Mark, 45 years old: Mark had been overweight, having trouble sleeping, and having high blood pressure for many years. Mark started sleeping better after we gave him a CPAP machine to treat his sleep apnea. He also lost weight, had better blood pressure, and had a lower risk of having more heart problems.

Accepting Sleep as a Key Part of Heart Health
They show how sleep can be very good for your heart in the stories of Sarah, Carlos, Linda, and Mark. However, sleep is often one of the least thought about aspects of heart health, even though it is very important. Many people worry about what they eat and how much they

exercise, but they forget how important rest is for keeping their hearts healthy.

It's time to accept that sleep is an important part of heart health. You give your heart the chance to heal and get stronger by making good sleep a priority. If you want to avoid heart disease or take care of a condition you already have, getting better sleep can help you in many ways, from lowering your blood pressure to making you feel better mentally and physically.

You can change your sleep habits for the better, whether you're having trouble sleeping right now or just want to keep your heart healthy.

After thinking about it, Sarah's journey from not being able to sleep to better heart health shows how important rest is for heart health. She learned that sleep wasn't just a nice to have, but a heart healthy must. Like Sarah, anyone can make changes that will help them sleep better and make their heart stronger for years to come.

CONCLUSION

Stronger Live And Longer Life

As we come to the end of this journey, I want to leave you with one last thought, how well you rest has a big impact on your health, vitality, and longevity. We've learned a lot about the strong link between sleep and heart health in this book. If you want to live a longer, healthier life, you can't ignore this link.

Restful sleep is not a privilege, it is a must if you want to get your health back. Similarly, your heart works hard for you, and it's your job to give it the rest it needs to heal. Putting your sleep first is the first step to better heart health, whether you're stressed, have a sleep problem, or just need to change some habits.

Getting Your Health Back Through Rest

The ideas and suggestions in this book have given you the tools to change the way you sleep, lower your risk of heart problems, and improve your general health. When it comes to heart health, not having heart disease, being tired, and having energy, getting more sleep can really make a difference.

It's time to act now. Use the tips you've learned to get better sleep. Prioritize rest, and see how your body reacts by getting stronger and more alive.

A Roadmap to Lifelong Heart Health

You can keep your heart healthy for life if you get enough sleep. From now on, look at every night as a chance to heal, restore, and protect your heart. Sleep should be the base on which your health is built.

Now that you know what to do, do it. Get enough rest, live a healthy life, and enjoy it.

A good night's sleep is all that stands between you and a better, longer life.